I0436975

Little Secrets

Little Secrets

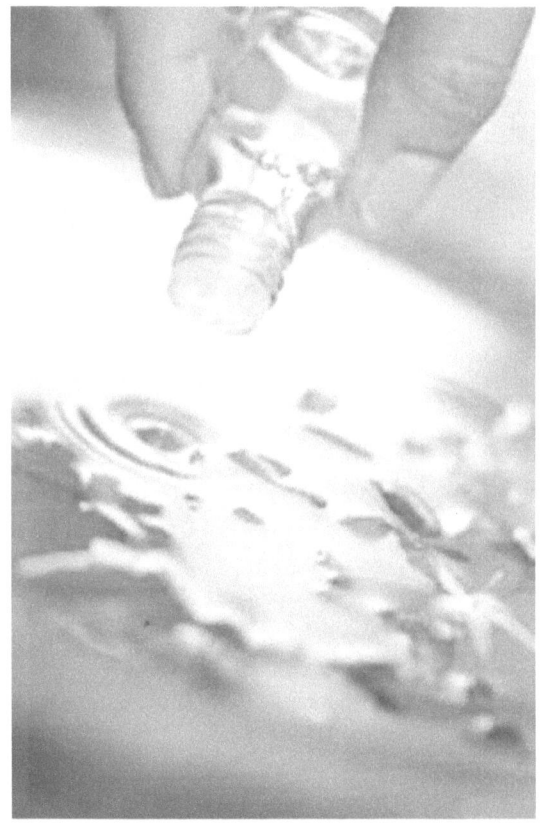

Lorie Bennett

Copyright © 2012 by Lorie Bennett.

ISBN: Softcover   978-1-4771-4730-6
                 Ebook   978-1-4771-4731-3

All rights reserved. No part of this book may be reproduced or transmitted in any form or by any means, electronic or mechanical, including photocopying, recording, or by any information storage and retrieval system, without permission in writing from the copyright owner.

This book was printed in the United States of America.

To order additional copies of this book, contact:
Xlibris Corporation
1-888-795-4274
www.Xlibris.com
Orders@Xlibris.com
119890

CREDITS

Author's Photograph: by Eric Bennett

Disclaimer/Warning:

Please ensure that you are NOT allergic to any of the products/ ingredients in the recipes prior to using them. Do NOT risk using these recipes if you believe you might have an allergic reaction. I am NOT a medical professional but I choose to use these ingredients/products as written. If you use these recipes, you do so at your own discretion without liability to anyone involved in the making of this book.

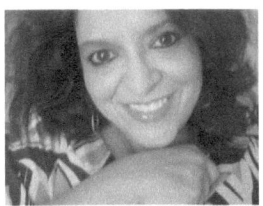

A WORD FROM THE AUTHOR

Thanks to everyone who helped make this book another reality for me. Even as an author, it is never taken for granted that another book has been published. I'm humbled and grateful to God for the opportunities given to me. I take nothing for granted.

To my family and friends; I love you!

To my lifelong friend—P.S. you know.

I hope you enjoy this DIY book. Use what has been given to me over the years and enjoy these recipes. Thanks to my "mom" who preached taking care of my skin since I was fifteen years old! I was given recipes, tricks and remedies that I am now able to pass on to you. These are not all my personal recipes; they have been shared with me. But they will make you feel pampered. Use the recipes as written or get creative and put your own spin on them; I did! Either way, you will save money and make a good product. I hope you enjoy my "feel good" book of *Little Secrets*.

Living overseas, one tends to pick up on a few things. While learning the beautiful European culture, I learned a new word "Tschuess". It has become my favorite word to use as an informal good-bye. So, to my new readers and my not so new . . .

Remember *". . . there's always something better, but this works too!"*

Tschuess! ☺

-Lorie

CONTENTS

Lets' Talk:

Natural healing takes time. And that is exactly what many of these products do—heal. So, if used daily, these products will show improvement and do exactly what I claim that they can do. These recipes have been used for centuries, but many of these recipes have my personal twist. If you use store made ingredients; it's okay, but then it won't be considered "all natural" in most cases. It won't change the outcome. Just keep that in mind as you browse through the recipes. The ingredients should be harmless—but make sure you are not allergic prior to using. The results that these recipes will give you are temporary; only surgery will result in a more permanent solution. Feel free to revise and add your own spin to these recipes. By adding more than the recipe calls for, it will give you a greater quantity.

I wanted this to be a "fun" book. I wrote it the way I would actually make the products. It's not the typical DIY book you will normally find. I put my personal spin, results and "two cents" on them. Enjoy and experiment. If you use these recipes on a regular basis and include them in your daily routine—the results are phenomenal. Pick a few and stick with them! You will want to make this a part of your daily routine after you see and feel the results. By using these products, you can and will save money. Plus, it's fun to make things and call them your own!

I am not a medical professional. It is best to check with your doctor prior to starting any new regime. I use these products and they have been effective for me. I hope you will have the same results and that you enjoy them. These are fun recipes that yield good results if used regularly!

Now on to the recipes . . . .

MEASUREMENTS

BASICS AT A GLANCE

Recipe Abbreviations

approx. = approximate
tsp or t = teaspoon
Tbsp or T = tablespoon
c = cup
pt = pint
qt = quart
gal = gallon
wt = weight
oz = ounce
lb or # = pound (e.g., 3#)

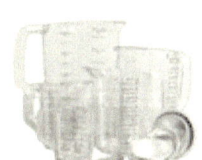

Volume Equivalents for Liquids

60 drops = 1 tsp
1 Tbsp = 3 tsp = 0.5 fl oz
1/8 cup = 2 Tbsp = 1 fl oz
1/4 cup = 4 Tbsp = 2 fl oz
1/3 cup = 5 Tbsp + 1 tsp = 2.65 fl oz
3/8 cup = 6 Tbsp = 3 fl oz
1/2 cup = 8 Tbsp = 4 fl oz
5/8 cup = 10 Tbsp = 5 fl oz
2/3 cup = 10 Tbsp + 2 tsp = 5.3 fl oz
3/4 cup = 12 Tbsp = 6 fl oz
7/8 cup = 14 Tbsp = 7 fl oz
1 cup = 16 Tbsp = 8 fl oz

TIP: Keeping product refrigerated prolongs the product.

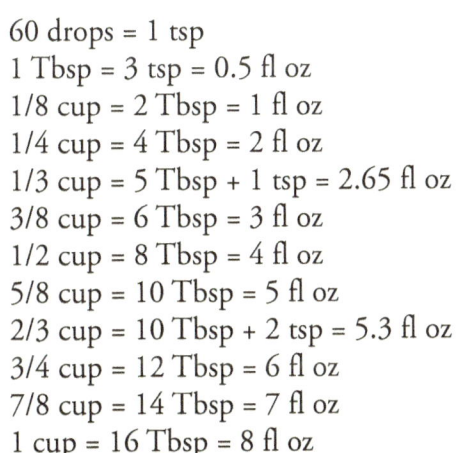
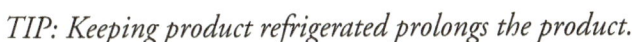

FACE

FACE MASK

Ingredients:

1 bowl
Wipes/tissues
1 egg white (whip)
1 t honey
1 t Glycerin

Recipe and Routine:

Mix all ingredients. (Store bought items okay to use). You do not need raw honey or vegetable glycerin. (Whichever you choose to use, will work.) Rub mask all over face. Put enough to leave a thick coating on your face. Leave for 20 minutes. Rinse with warm water. Wipe face clean. Use once a week for best results.

Uses:

Use for anti-wrinkle and moisturizer.

SETTING SPRAY

Ingredients:

1 spray bottle
1 part Glycerin
3 parts Spring (or Distilled) water
2 pumps Aloe Gel

Recipe and Routine:

Mix 1 part glycerin with 3 parts spring water; shake. Add 2 pumps of aloe gel (any brand). You can use the cap of the glycerin bottle as your measuring tool. Whatever you choose to use, make sure it's a 1:3 ratio.

Uses:

Spray on daily after applying makeup. Sets makeup for all day results. Makes your foundation smooth; not cakey. TIP: If used with powder foundation, it will give you a glowy appearance. Use with eyeshadow for a vibrant tint. Use during summer for a face spritz and to freshen makeup during the day.

TINTED SPRAY

Ingredients:

1 spray bottle
1 part Glycerin
3 parts Spring (or Distilled) water
2 pumps Aloe Gel
2 T body butter of choice
2 T foundation (any color)

Recipe and Routine:

Mix 1 part glycerin with 3 parts spring water; shake. Add 2 pumps of aloe gel (any brand). You can use the cap of the glycerin bottle as your measuring tool. Whatever you choose to use, make sure it's a 1:3 ratio. Add the body butter and foundation to the mix. Shake, shake, shake!

Uses:

Spray on daily. Can be used in place of heavier makeup on a summer day. If you do use foundation over this, the spray serves as a primer. Sets makeup for all day results.

PORE STRIPS

Ingredients:

1 microwaveable bowl
1 T unflavored boxed Jello powder
1 T Milk

Recipe and Routine:

Stir all ingredients together. Stir until nice and chunky! Microwave for 10 seconds to ensure it has a sticky consistency. Let cool. Apply to nose. Wait until completely dry. Then gently take a corner and peel off the strip.

Uses:

This serves to clean out pores and strip away blackheads.

TINTED MOISTURIZER

Ingredients:

1 resealable bowl
1 body butter of choice
1 T Glycerin
1 T foundation (any color)
1 T SPF lotion (your choice)

Recipe and Routine:

Mix all ingredients. (Store bought items—okay to use.) Any color foundation is acceptable because the mixture will make it very light and it will not show up on the face the way it does in non-diluted form.

Uses:

Used for moisturizer and serves as a primer.

1 STEP MASK

Ingredients:

1 resealable bowl
1 container of Plain Yogurt
1 brush (makeup or soft paint brush)

Recipe and Routine:

Open jar and put a generous amount on the brush. Paint your face with the yogurt. Repeat until face is fully coated. Make sure you have a thick coat. Let dry for about 20 minutes (longer, if necessary). Rinse with warm water.

Uses:

Benefit is that it will serve as a hydrating mask and also cleanse the skin. Caution: This can be used around the eyes, but be careful because it does sting if it gets into your eyes. If that happens, rinse with cool water.

MATURE SKIN ROUTINE

Ingredients:

1 bowl
1 bowl of warm water or stand by sink
1 face towel
3 T Olive Oil (your choice)

Recipe and Routine:

Wet towel with warm water. Dip towel in Olive Oil. Take soaked portion and gently rub over face in circular motions. This will exfoliate your face. Gently rinse face with warm water. If you desire, mild facial soap can be used. TIP: It can be used all over your body in the shower for full body exfoliation.

Uses:

Used for exfoliation and as a skin moisturizer.

FACE EXFOLIATOR

Ingredients:

1-3 Uncoated Aspirins
1 small container or hands

Recipe and Routine:

Dissolve aspirins with warm water. Gently rub face with finger or cloth. While in the shower, hold aspirins in your hand as you would with liquid soap or pour from the container where you put your mixture. This can be made in a larger quantity for full body use. It does not store well, so it is best to use the same day that you make it.

Uses:

Use once a week. This is used for exfoliation.

MOISTURIZER

Ingredients:

1 bowl
1 spoon of Petroleum Jelly (your choice)
1 face towel
1 cotton swab

Recipe and Routine:

Wet towel with warm water. Let towel be wet, but not dripping. Dip towel in Petroleum Jelly. Take soaked portion and gently rub over face avoiding eyes. This will moisturize your face.

Uses:

Used as a diluted skin moisturizer. Best if used at night. This method allows for the face to absorb product and soften the skin. This works best on dry skin. You can put this on troubled areas such as the "T-zone". Caution: Best to avoid this method if you have acne prone skin.

ACNE TONER

Ingredients:

3 Uncoated Aspirins
½ bottle of Witch Hazel
1 bottle

Recipe and Routine:

Pour Witch Hazel half way into the container being used. Dissolve aspirins in Witch Hazel (drop them into the bottle opening). Shake vigorously. Once aspirins have dissolved, mixture will be cloudy. Take a cotton swab and dab over clean face. Best for both morning and night routines. Use daily.

Uses:

This is used for toning the skin. Pores will gradually get smaller. This method helps with acne prone skin. It will not reduce signs of scars, but will help control outbreaks.

TONER

Ingredients:

1 bottle of Witch Hazel
1 cotton swab

Recipe and Routine:

Pour Witch Hazel onto a cotton swab. Rub all over clean face in an upward motion.

Uses:

Used as a facial toner. This method works best on normal skin. Product can be a bit drying, but if used sparingly, it is a great product. Other uses include sun burn, hiding blood vessels (shrinks them), bug bites and much more. It does not have a very pleasant odor. If this is too bothersome, put 1-2 drops of Essence Oil for scent.

TOOTHPASTE

Ingredients:

3 T Baking Soda
1 T Sea Salt
1T Glycerin
1-3 drops Fruit Essential Oil (i.e., cinnamon/mint)

Recipe and Routine:

Mix. Recipe should be sticky. Shake if necessary, then store. If you like your toothpaste runny and not so sticky—cut back on the baking soda until you get desired consistency. Store in bathroom. TIP: For flavored toothpaste you can add sweetener or drops of flavoring.

Uses:

Used to clean teeth and gum areas.

LIP BALM

Ingredients:

1 tube or jar with lid (microwave safe)
1 stir stick/spoon
1 T Vaseline
1-3 drops fruit oil scent
1 scrape of eyeshadow (your choice color) OR
1 scrape of lipstick (your choice color)

Recipe and Routine:

To make a tinted balm, mix in either eyeshadow or lipstick until you get the desired color. Color will be much lighter than what you see. This is just a conditioning balm. TIP: Leave the color out of the recipe and you can make clear balm. Add all products to the mix with stir stick. Mix well and quickly to prevent settling. Microwave for 30 seconds. (Microwave time may vary. This will melt it down so that when it freezes, it is nice and smooth!) Freeze 10 minutes. Ready to use.

Uses:

Used as a moisturizer for your lips. (Time may vary according to freezer and microwave settings, but the end result should be the same regardless of time adjustments.)

LIP BALM (FLAVORED)

Ingredients:

1 tube or jar with lid (microwave safe)
1 T Aquaphor
1 T Vaseline
2 t Crystal Light (prepared) OR Kool-Aid (your choice color and flavor)

Recipe and Routine:

Fill bowl with ingredients. Color will be much lighter than what you see. Mix well and quickly to prevent settling. Microwave for 30 seconds. (Microwave time may vary. This will melt it down so that when it freezes, it is nice and smooth!) Freeze 10 minutes. Ready to use.

Uses:

Used as a moisturizer for your lips. (Time may vary according to freezer and microwave settings, but the end result should be the same regardless of time adjustments.) The tint will not be a vibrant color, but serves more for the flavoring in your lip balm.

LORIE BENNETT

MOUTHWASH

Ingredients:

1 c Distilled/Spring water
2 T Glycerin
2 drops Essential Oil (i.e., cinnamon, mint, orange)

Recipe and Routine:

Mix ingredients in a bottle; shake well. Store at room temperature. Rinse mouth when needed.

Uses:

This is used for a mouth rinse. If swallowed, no problem!

EYES

EYELASHES GROW

Ingredients:

1 clean and sterile mascara tube or Q-tip
1-3 drops of Olive Oil

Recipe and Routine:

Clean an old tube of mascara. Rinse, sterilize and rinse again. When water is clear, tube is cleaned inside. Dip your Q-tip or mascara brush into the olive oil. Gently apply as if you were putting on an application of mascara. Do this twice a day; every day. In about 2 weeks, you should see hair growth. If you have long eyelashes, this will keep them conditioned.

Uses:

Used for a moisturizer for the lashes. Best if used twice a day. Safe to use on upper and lower lids. This method allows for hair to stay moist and conditioned.

EYELASHES CONDITIONED

Ingredients:

1 clean and sterile mascara tube or Q-tip
1-3 drops of Castor Oil

Recipe and Routine:

Clean an old tube of mascara. Rinse, sterilize and rinse again. When water is clear, tube is cleaned inside. Dip your Q-tip or mascara brush into the castor oil. Gently apply as if you were putting on an application of mascara. Do this twice a day; every day. In about 2 weeks, you should experience less breakage. If you have long eyelashes, this will keep them conditioned.

Uses:

Used for a moisturizer for the lashes. Best if used twice a day. Safe to use on upper and lower lids. This method allows for hair to stay moist and conditioned. Some claim that it promotes eyelash hair growth.

EYE PRIMER

Ingredients:

1 T concealor, any color
3 T Glycerin
1 T Aloe Gel
1 mixing tool
1 container with lid

Recipe and Routine:

Mix all ingredients. Ready to use when all ingredients are mixed. Store at room temperature.

Uses:

Used for a moisturizer. Primes eyelids. Helps eye shadow and eyeliner last all day. Helps prevent the "eye shadow crease" that forms after all day wear.

HAND & NAIL

HAND MASK

Ingredients:

1 bowl
1 plastic bag
1 T sugar (granulated)
2 T Olive Oil
1 wipe

Recipe and Routine:

Mix ingredients together in a bowl. Gently rub mask all over hands. Make sure that you have a good solid layer. Put your hands in a plastic bag (baggie or plastic grocery bag works). Try to make sure that it is secure enough to allow heat to build up. Keep mask on for 15 minutes. Unwrap hands, clean hands with wipe, but do not rinse. Treat yourself to this mask at least once a month!

Uses:

Used for a moisturizer for hands and a conditioner for the nails and cuticles.

HAND TREATMENT

Ingredients:

1 bowl
Microwave
1 towel
½ cup heavy cream

Recipe and Routine:

Pour heavy cream into a bowl large enough to fit your fingertips. Microwave for 45 seconds. Let stand until cream is warm, not HOT. Then, dip your fingertips into the cream for 15 minutes. Relax! TIP: Added benefit if you rub your hands with the cream as you soak. Run warm water over hands to rinse. Gently dry. Moisturize with your favorite hand lotion or the lotion you make yourself!

Uses:

Used for a moisturizer for hands.

CUTICLE CONDITIONER

Ingredients:

1-2 Vitamin E caplets
1 needle

Recipe and Routine:

Puncture vitamin E pill. Squeeze and apply to cuticle area. Let stand and dry. Do not rinse. Best if applied at night or after morning routine so that it will stay on your hands until dry. Easy!

Uses:

Used for a moisturizer for the cuticles. You can use this as a nightly routine to prevent dryness and those "pesky" cuticles that pop up and get caught in stockings or stick up making hands look unkept! TIP: Some users claim that by keeping cuticles groomed and moisturized that it promotes nail growth!

HAND AGE SPOT LIGHTENER

Ingredients:

1 clean towel, soft cloth or cotton swab
1-3 drops of Castor Oil

Recipe and Routine:

Gently rub an application of castor oil to the top of your hand. Let dry.

Uses:

After extended use, age spots will begin to lighten. This is not a bleaching agent and will not bleach your skin. By adding moisture to the age spots, it gives the appearance of lighter spots.

LIGHTEN AGE SPOTS

Ingredients:

½ lemon
½ T sugar

Recipe and Routine:

Rub lemon juice on hand. Make sure you do not have open cuts/wounds. Take sugar and sprinkle on top of hand. Gently rub in circular motion. The sugar may dissolve, but you do not have to rub until it is completely dissolved. Do this for 2 minutes (1 minute per hand), then wipe clean.

Uses:

After extended use, age spots will begin to lighten. This does serve as a *mild* bleaching agent. It will not harm your skin, but can lighten. Be sure to moisturize once you use this method to keep the moisture in the hand even and equal throughout the hand.

SOAP

Ingredients:

1 goat milk soap base
1 color (dye) brick (drops also available)
Scent (your choice of oil)
Knife
Ladle
Plastic mold
Crock pot

Recipe and Routine:

Pour ingredients into the crock pot (LOW heat). Add dye brick-leave until it turns the color that you like. Add 1 capful of scent. When mixture is completely melted, drop liquid into mold. Let stand for 6 hours. Ready to use.

Uses:

This is a very easy method. It is commonly referred to as the "melt and pour" method. This is not a complicated recipe, but it works!

FEET

SOFT FEET

Ingredients:

1 pair of socks
1 scoop Vaseline

Recipe and Routine:

With your hands, gently apply a generous amount of Vaseline on feet. Concentrate on dry areas. Put socks on your feet. Best to use at night. TIP: If you do not like to sleep with socks on, follow this same routine, but put your feet in a plastic bag for 1 hour. Same results!

Uses:

Used as a moisturizer for feet. Best if used daily; especially in "sandal" weather! Using this method on a regular basis will help to keep dry feet moisturized.

FOOT SOAK

Ingredients:

1 c Olive Oil
¼ c Sea Salt
1 large bowl

Recipe and Routine:

Mix ingredients in bowl. Place feet in the bowl and soak for 30 minutes (or longer). Remove feet from foot soak; pat dry.

Uses:

Used as a moisturizer for your feet, but also helps with exfoliation. Best if used on a regular basis.

HAIR

HAIR SPRITZ

Ingredients:

4 oz Distilled water
3 oz Glycerin
2 squirts Aloe Gel
1-3 drops Essential Oil (optional)
3 T conditioner (any will do)
1 bottle

Recipe and Routine:

Mix and spritz!

Uses:

Used as a moisturizer for your hair. This can be used any time, all day, every day. The concept is the same as a "leave in moisturizer". Can be used on any hair type and color/processed hair.

HAIR SHINE

Ingredients:

2 T Sea Salt
1 spray bottle
1 c Distilled (or Spring) water

Recipe and Routine:

Fill bottle ¼ of the way with distilled water. Add sea salt to bottle. Shake vigorously. Spray on dry hair.

Uses:

This recipe is easy and harmless. It makes your hair shiny without the heavy oil in most shine sprays. This is a temporary shine; but it will not bleach or damage your hair. Can be used on any hair type.

HAIR LIGHTENER

Ingredients:

1 oz Lemon juice (concentrate)
2 oz Conditioner (your choice)
3 oz Distilled water
1 spray bottle
1 plastic bag

Recipe and Routine:

Fill bottle with all ingredients. Mix product. Spray on areas where you want lighter hair (hi-lights.) No need to rinse. Style as normal. TIP: You can spray on dry hair and go!

Uses:

This recipe is easy and harmless. It makes your hair lighter without harsh chemicals. It does take time, but it works. The more exposure to the sun, the faster it works (while product is on hair). It is temporary, but safe to use with dyed hair.

HAIR LIGHTENER

Ingredients:

2 oz Honey (raw or store bought)
2 oz Conditioner (your choice)
1 spray or regular bottle
1 plastic bag

Recipe and Routine:

Fill bottle with all ingredients. Mix product. Apply on areas where you want lighter hair. Leave on for 30 minutes with hair wrapped in plastic bag. Rinse. Style as normal.

Uses:

This recipe is easy and harmless. It makes your hair lighten without harsh chemicals. It does take time. But over the course of a few weeks, you will have highlights where you have applied your lightener. It is temporary, but will not damage your hair.

SHAMPOO

Ingredients:

Measuring cup
Reuse empty shampoo bottle
Castile Liquid soap
2 oz Olive Oil
Distilled water (amount depends on bottle size)

Recipe and Routine:

Fill bottle ¼ of the way with Castile Liquid Soap. (Any will do, but I use Dr. Bronner's Pure Castile Soap with Lavender Oil). Fill bottle with olive oil and fill bottle up with remaining water ingredient. Shake. Use. Style as normal.

Uses:

This recipe is easy and harmless. The "suds" are pretty close to store bought brands. This is an easy way to make shampoo that works. TIP: Add some Bay essential oil to help with dandruff!

HAIR SPRAY

Ingredients:

½ lemon (cut into quarters—do not peel)
2 oranges (cut into 4 sections—do not peel)
2 c Distilled/bottled water
1 pot
1 spray bottle

Recipe and Routine:

Boil water with the fruit, in the pan (peeling and all). MEDIUM heat. Bring to boil. Cover for 10 minutes. Strain ingredients into the bottle of choice (spray bottle). Chill product for 1 hour. Use.

Uses:

This recipe is easy and harmless. It offers a light hold. The oranges make it "hold". That is the secret to this recipe! Safe for all hair types.

CONDITION MASK

Ingredients:

1 egg
4 T Olive Oil
3 scoops Mayonnaise (real)
1 plastic bag
1 bottle

Recipe and Routine:

Mix and spread all over hair. Concentrate on the ends of your hair and work upward. Cover your head with plastic bag (any will do). Cover for 30 minutes for a deep conditioning effect. Rinse.

Uses:

Used as a moisturizer for your hair.

BODY

CONDITIONING BATH SCRUB

Ingredients:

1 bowl
1 c Coconut Oil (melted)
1 T Jojoba Oil
1 T Vitamin C
1 T Vitamin E
2 T Olive Oil
1 c Sugar (granulated)
1-3 drops Essential Oil (optional)

Recipe and Routine:

Melt coconut oil, then let cool. Mix all remaining ingredients. Combine. Let sit 1 hour. Pour into container with lid. Store in bathtub or bathroom. Use in shower daily.

Uses:

Gently exfoliates with the sugar added. No need to use lotion afterwards!

NATURAL DETOX DRINK

Ingredients:

1 beet
4 carrots
½ cucumber

Recipe and Routine:

Blend with mixer or blender into a smoothie texture. Chill for 1 hour. Drink.

Uses:

This is a natural detox drink. There is no water used in this drink. If it is too strong for you and you do not like the texture or flavor; add ½ cup of water. It will not change the effectiveness. Safe to drink daily, but if you do not have bowel movement issues; once or twice a month is enough.

DEORDANT

Ingredients:

1 bowl
8 oz jar with lid or old dispenser
¼ c Baking Soda
¼ c Corn Starch
6 T Coconut Oil

Recipe and Routine:

Fill bowl with all powder ingredients. Incorporate coconut oil into mixture. Continue to mix (adding more if necessary) until the consistency is like cookie dough. Doing this with a spoon or your hand works best. A mixer works, but it makes it too runny. TIP: Add 2 drops of peppermint or tea tree essential oil for a unisex scent! Gently fill jar or old Deordant dispenser with product. Apply on underarm area.

Uses:

This recipe is easy and harmless. It is an effective recipe for homemade Deordant. The essential oil gives a pleasant aroma for men or women. If you use an old Deordant container, the product will not get all over your hands. It is safe to apply with fingertips though! Store at room temperature.

BODY LOTION

Ingredients:

Set stove on MEDIUM heat
1 pan with 2 c tap water
2 bowls
1 GLASS measuring cup
1 ½ c Distilled water
¼ c Emulsified Wax
¼ c Olive Oil
1 bottle

Recipe and Routine:

Put pan with water on stovetop. Place measuring cup into the pan and fill measuring cup with wax and olive oil. Stir until melted. Heat 1 bowl with distilled water in microwave or (on stove) for 2 minutes. Pour heated water and mixture of wax and olive oil together. (It looks like skim milk.) Pour combined mixture into the bottle to store lotion. Cool 1 hour, then use. Complete all steps prior to storing!

Uses:

Body lotion made easy. If you add 3 drops of Vitamin E oil or one capsule (punctured) it will add shelf life to your product. Add a few drops of essential oil for scent.

WEBSITES & MORE

WEBSITES TO ORDER PRODUCTS:

Drugstore.com
Amazon.com
Ebay.com
Iherb.com
Newdirectionsaromatics.com
Localharvest.org

STORES TO BUY CONTAINERS AND PRODUCTS:

Health Food Stores
Grocery Stores
Walmart
Target
K Mart
Dollar General
99 Cent store
Michael's

NOTES:

Remember to sterilize all containers. Rinse with alcohol; it's that easy! (Especially important tip for those products on your face.)

My roommate/friend used to poke fun at me with, "You can never leave the house without eyeliner". And that I should invest in whatever brand I was using at the time. She was right; I never leave the house without eyeliner. However, I still have to buy it since I haven't figured out how to make it!!" ☺

This book gives you some ideas on how to DIY your own products, but I haven't figured out how to make everything. These websites and store suggestions will give you a chance to tap into your creative side. Check all your favorite shopping areas. You'll be surprised where these products are available! And even though you still have to purchase store bought products; I know you will save money!

ESSENTIAL OILS & THEIR HEALING PROPERTIES (SHORT VERSION)

ESSENCE	PHYSICAL	EMOTIONAL (helps with)
Angelica Root	Dull skin, gout	nervousness, stress, exhaustion
Anise	Bronchitis, colds, flatulence	depression
Basil	Bronchitis, colds, insect bites	fatigue, exhaustion, concentration
Bay	Dandruff, oily skin, poor circulation	exhaustion, fatigue
Bay Laurel	loss of appetite, tonsils tonsillitis	mental confusion, confidence
Benzoin	arthritis, bronchitis,	chapped skin insecurity
Bergamot	acne, abscess, anxiety, itching	anger, anxiety, confidence
Rosewood	acne, colds, scars, stretch marks, dry skin, sensitive skin	depression, emotional imbalance
Cajuput	Asthma, aches, sinus	confusion, fatigue
Cardamom	appetite loss, colic, halitosis	fatigue, shame guilt
Carrot seed	Eczema, mature skin, toxins	anxiety, confusion, mood swings
Cedarwood	Acne, arthritis, dermatitis	fear, insecurity, stress
Chamomile	Allergies, arthritis, cuts, stress	anger, anxiety, depression, PMS
Cinnamon	Constipation, flatulence, lice, LBP	emotional, mental fatigue, concentration
Citronella	Insect repellent, oily skin, sweating	mind fog, tension
Elemi	Bronchitis, cough, mature skin	agitation, grief

Clary Sage	labor pains, sore throat	loneliness, stress, anxiety
Coriander	aches, arthritis, colic, indigestion	irritation
Cypress	perspiration, varicose veins	confidence, concentration
Eucalyptus	arthritis, cold sore, sinus	agitation, grief
Fennel	Bruises, cellulite, gums	emotional imbalance, fatigue
Frankincense	Stretch marks, scars, bronchitis	burnout, panic attack, anxiety
Galbanum	immune system, abscess, wounds	rigidity, mood swings, nervousness
Geranium	Acne, cellulite, dull skin, lice	anxiety, depression, mood imbalance
Ginger	Aching muscles, arthritis	fatigue exhaustion, burnout
Grapefruit	Water retention, toxins, dull skin	peace, stress, confidence

ESSENCE	PHYSICAL	EMOTIONAL (helps with)
Helichryseum	abscess, boils, cuts, wound	exhaustion, panic, shock
Hyssop	bruises, cough, sore throat	concentration, nervousness
Jasmine	dry skin, labor pains, skin	depression, exhaustion, anger
Juniper Berry	cellulite, hemorrhoids, obesity	agitation, negative emotions
Lavender	acne, allergy, asthma, chicken pox	depression, irritability, panic attacks
Lemon	athlete's foot, corns, spots, varicose veins	stress, panic attacks, tension
Lemongrass	acne, digestion, scabies, skin	fatigue, mental confusion
Linden Blossom	headache, migraines, wrinkles	insomnia, stress, tension
Marjoram	aching muscles, cramps	mood swings, PMS, stress
Melissa	flu indigestion, herpes, nausea	agitation, anxiety dementia
Myrrh	athlete's foot, bronchitis, chapped skin	creativity, imbalanced moods
Myrtle	acne, irritated skin	addition, self destructive behavior

Neroli	mature skin, stretch marks	stress, panic attacks, anxiety
Niauoli	acne, bronchitis, cold, cough	concentration and mental fog
Nutmeg	constipation, poor circulation	mental fatigue
Bitter Orange	constipation, flu, gums, mouth	anger, depression, stress
Oregano	digestion, respiration	insecurity
Parsley	digestion, diuretic, immune system	frigidity
Pepper (Black)	aching muscles, detox, cramps, poor circulation	anxiety, fatigue, concentration
Peppermint asthma, sinus, nausea, vertigo	memory, concentration, exhaustion	
Pine	colds, congestion, flu	depression, nervous exhaustion
Rose	eczema, mature skin	anger, anxiety, menopause, stress
Sandalwood	bronchitis, skin, laryngitis, oily skin	depression, fear, grief, irritability
Spearmint	asthma, headache, nausea	depression, mental fatigue
Thyme	arthritis, bronchitis, cuts	concentration and memory

For an in depth list search the Internet for "essence oils and their properties"

INGREDIENTS AND THEIR BENEFITS
(SHORT VERSION)

Aloe	heals, antibacterial, natural preservative
Baking Soda	gently exfoliates, eliminates odors
Castor Oil	disinfecting properties
Cornstarch	purity, thickens
Eggs	contain essential nutrients
Glycerin	lubricating, soothing, emollient
Green Tea	antioxidant, soothing
Honey	breaks down easily, not harsh
Mayonnaise	oil, moisturizer
Olive Oil	antioxidant, vitamins, moisturizing
Sea Salt	exfoliates breaks down easily
Tea tree	antibacterial, antifungal
Vaseline	replicates paraffin treatment, relief of dry skin
Vinegar	removes residues, freshens
Vitamin C	anti-aging properties
Vitamin E	natural preservative, heals
Witch Hazel	heals, protects, cleanses
Yogurt	refreshes, moisturizes

For an in depth list search the Internet for "ingredients and their health benefits" or type in the ingredient name for specific information.

www.ingramcontent.com/pod-product-compliance
Lightning Source LLC
Chambersburg PA
CBHW020353290526
45785CB00005B/2256